THE FINA AND APPETIZERS COOKBOOK

Inspire your vegan cooking desire with these 50 kitchen-tested recipes

Laura Mckinney

© **Copyright 2021 by Jordan Editors - All rights reserved.**

The following Book is reproduced below with the goal of providing information that is as accurate and reliable as possible. Regardless, purchasing this Book can be seen as consent to the fact that both the publisher and the author of this book are in no way experts on the topics discussed within and that any recommendations or suggestions that are made herein are for entertainment purposes only. Professionals should be consulted as needed prior to undertaking any of the action endorsed herein.

This declaration is deemed fair and valid by both the American Bar Association and the Committee of Publishers Association and is legally binding throughout the United States. Furthermore, the transmission, duplication, or reproduction of any of the following work including specific information will be considered an illegal act irrespective of if it is done electronically or in print. This extends to creating a secondary or tertiary copy of the work or a recorded copy and is only allowed with the express written consent from the Publisher. All additional right reserved.

The information in the following pages is broadly considered a truthful and accurate account of facts and as such, any inattention, use, or misuse of the information in question by the reader will render any resulting actions solely under their purview. There are no scenarios in which the publisher or the original author of this work can be in any fashion deemed liable for any hardship or damages that may befall them after undertaking information described herein.

Additionally, the information in the following pages is intended only for informational purposes and should thus be thought of as universal. As befitting its nature, it is presented without assurance regarding its prolonged validity or interim quality. Trademarks that are mentioned are done without written consent and can in no way be considered an endorsement from the trademark holder.

Table of contents

THE FINAL VEGAN SNACKS AND APPETIZERS COOKBOOK 1

© COPYRIGHT 2021 BY JORDAN EDITORS - ALL RIGHTS RESERVED. 2

TABLE OF CONTENTS... 4

INTRODUCTION 7

    BOILED PEANUTS 12
    TOFU WRAPS 13
    PUMPKIN HUMMUS 15
    ROASTED NUTS 17
    SPICY EDAMAME SNACK 19
    TEMPEH POTATO WRAPS 21
    VEGAN NUGGETS 23
    CRUNCHWRAP SUPREME 26
    SPRING ROLLS 28
    DELICIOUS LETTUCE WRAPS 30
    GARLIC TOASTS 32
    CRISPY CHICKPEA 34
    TURKISH VEGAN BOREK 37
    VEGAN JERKY 38
    CARROT "DOGS" 40
    GYROS 42
    HERBED TOMATO 44
    LENTILS CRACKERS 46
    EGGPLANT ROLLS 49
    MUSHROOM BRUSCHETTA 51
    BBQ CAULIFLOWER FLORETS 53
    ASPARAGUS PASTRIES 55
    COCKTAIL BALLS 58
    ARUGULA PUFFS 60
    BEETROOT FOLD-OVERS 62
    SWEET APPLE WEDGES 64
    CANDIED PECANS 66
    BUFFALO BRUSSEL SPROUTS 69
    MUSHROOM PATE 71
    CARDAMOM PINEAPPLE STICKS 73
    APPETIZER QUINOA BALLS 74
    TOFU STRIPS 74

CHICKPEA SLICES	78
CRUNCHY OYSTER MUSHROOMS	80
JACKFRUIT COATED BITES	82
SOFRITAS TOFU	84
GARLIC PUMPKIN SEEDS	86
FLATBREAD	87
POLENTA FRIES	88
GREEN CROQUETTES	90
CIGAR BOREK	92
FLAKED CLUSTERS	93
CHICKPEA CRACKERS	95
EGGPLANT FRIES	98
CRUNCHY ARTICHOKE HEARTS	100
SCALLION PANCAKES	101
MUSHROOM ARANCINI	103
COATED HEART OF PALM	105
SWEET TOFU CUBES	107

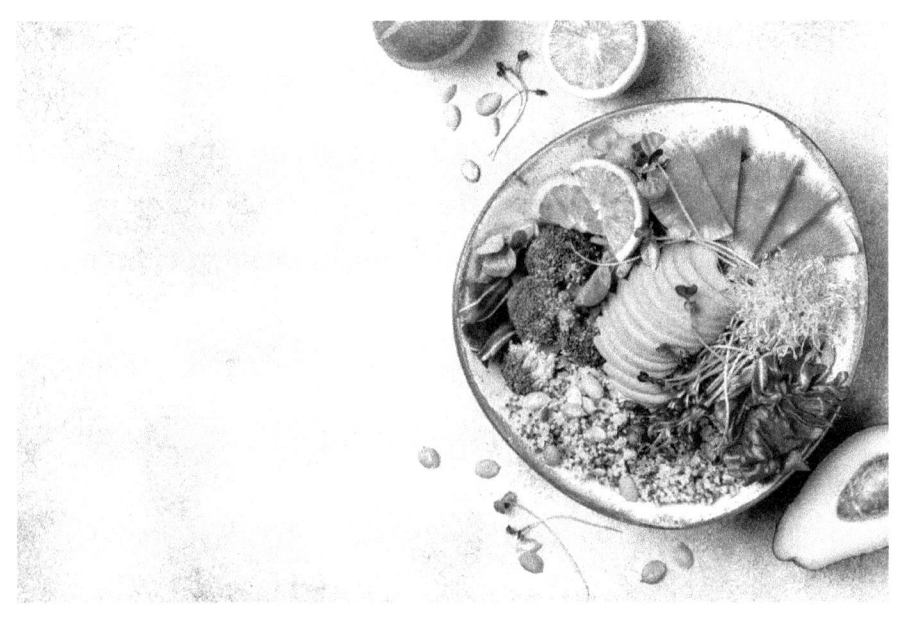

Introduction

Veganism is one of the most followed trends around the world today.
There are many people who have decided not to take more food products deriving from animal products and to follow a lifestyle in harmony with nature. The history of the vegan diet began in 1944 with a diet specially formulated for the purpose, five years later Leslie J Cross suggested the idea of veganism by supporting the idea of emancipating animals from human exploitation.
Over the years, veganism has become not only a food habit but a real lifestyle, influencing hundreds of thousands of people, for whom it shares an attitude of respect and protection of animals and nature in general.

Veganism involves the abolition of the diet of any food derived from meat, poultry, seafood, and dairy products. Contrary to what one might think, however, the vegan diet is very varied and full of succulent and very different dishes, to satisfy any preference. From breakfast to dinner you can vary to your liking with very good and satisfying sweet and savory dishes. The only condition is that each meal is made with ingredients of plant origin. And don't think that the vegan diet has limits on nutrients, because vitamins, minerals, and vital proteins can be taken from vegetables, fruits, cereals, nuts, and seeds. It will be enough to practice a little and the result will certainly be in line with our expectations, thanks also to an increasingly refined technology of cooking meals. Vegan food is very varied, from vegan ice cream, to burritos, cheese, burgers, mayonnaise and so much more. Being vegan does not mean depriving yourself of something, on the contrary, it means improving your lifestyle in harmony with the nature of which we are part.

The vegan diet also includes the consumption of lettuce, pasta, chips, bread, and various sauces.

The reasons that push people to become vague can be the most disparate, the lifestyle they assume certainly benefits everyone! The vegetable diet is sufficiently rich in iron, folic acid, magnesium, vitamins C and B1 which are essential for our body. At the same time, the vegan diet can never include a high amount of saturated fat and cholesterol.

Also, veganism has obvious health benefits, helping to prevent serious diseases such as stroke, type 2 diabetes, obesity, colon and prostate cancer, hypertension, and ischemic heart disease. There are no age preclusions to follow a vegan diet, however, we recommend greater attention to the daily meal ratio, to avoid nutritional deficiencies.

In this cookbook, you will find 50 delicious recipes that will make you want to get up in the morning. There are recipes for every taste, just follow our advice and you can make real culinary masterpieces. Forget the boredom of thinking about what to eat, this cookbook will give you the right inspiration.

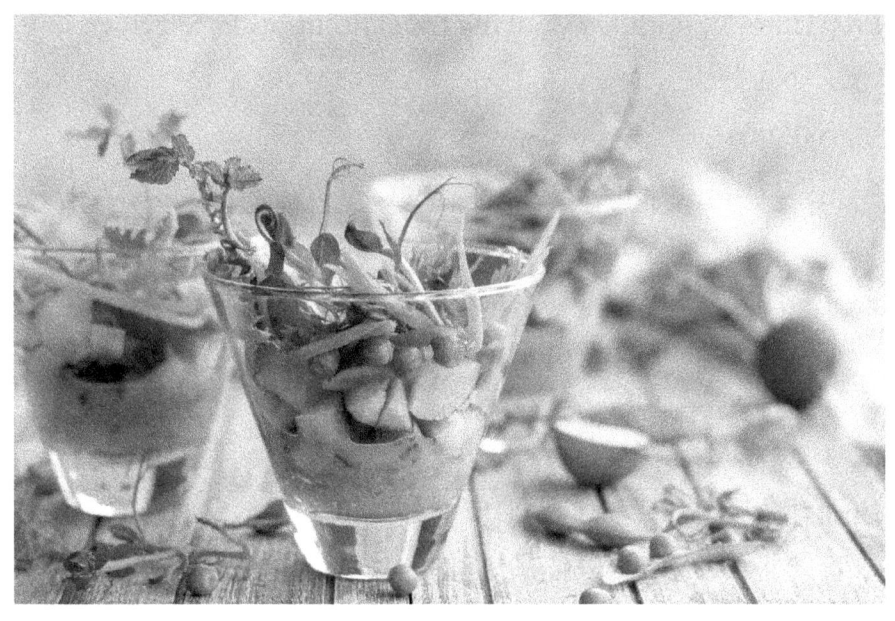

Boiled Peanuts

Prep time: 15 minutes Cooking time: 30 minutes Servings: 8

Ingredients:
- 2 cups green peanuts in shells
- 2 cups of water
- 2 teaspoons salt
- 1 teaspoon cayenne pepper
- 1 teaspoon taco seasoning

Directions:
14. Place green peanuts, water, salt, cayenne pepper, and taco seasoning in the instant pot.
15. Close the lid and set Manual mode (high pressure).
16. Cook the peanuts for 30 minutes.
17. When the time is over, allow natural pressure release for 10 minutes more.
18. Drain water and transfer peanuts in the serving bowl.

Nutrition value/serving: calories 168, fat 10.6, fiber 0.1, carbs 11.1, protein 7.5

Tofu Wraps

Prep time: 15 minutes Cooking time: 5 minutes Servings: 6

Ingredients:
- 6 lettuce leaves
- 1 teaspoon chili pepper
- 1 tablespoon fish sauce
- 1 teaspoon brown sugar
- 3 tablespoons water
- ½ teaspoon salt
- 8 oz firm tofu, chopped
- 1 teaspoon mustard
- 1 teaspoon olive oil
- 1 oz fresh curly parsley, chopped

Directions:
12. Make the tofu sauce: whisk together chili pepper, fish sauce, brown sugar, water, salt, mustard, and olive oil.
13. Then combine together tofu and sauce. Let it marinade for 10 minutes.
14. Preheat the instant pot on Saute mode well.
15. Place the tofu and all marinade inside; saute the ingredients for 5 minutes. Stir them from time to time.

16. When the time is over, open the instant pot lid and let tofu chill till the room temperature.
17. Fill the lettuce leaves with chopped parsley and tofu.
18. Before serving, sprinkle tofu wraps with the remaining cooked marinade.

Nutrition value/serving: calories 41, fat 2.6, fiber 0.7, carbs 2, protein 3.6

Pumpkin Hummus

Prep time: 10 minutes Cooking time: 45 minutes Servings: 6

Ingredients:
- ½ cup pumpkin puree
- 1 ½ chickpea, soaked
- 2 teaspoon tahini
- 1 teaspoon harissa
- 4 tablespoons olive oil
- 1 garlic clove, peeled
- 5 cups of water

Directions:
12. Place chickpeas and water in the instant pot.
13. Add garlic clove. Close and seal the lid.
14. Set Manual mode (high pressure) and cook chickpeas for 25 minutes.
15. When the time is over, allow natural pressure release for 20 minutes.
16. Open the lid and drain the liquid.
17. Transfer the cooked chickpeas and garlic clove in the food processor. Add pumpkin puree, tahini, harissa, and olive oil.

18. Blend the mixture until smooth and homogenous. If the cooked hummus is not soft enough, add water from the cooked chickpeas.

19. Store the cooked hummus in the fridge up to 3 days.

Nutrition value/serving: calories 212, fat 10.1, fiber 7.1, carbs 24.6, protein 7.7

Roasted Nuts

Prep time: 10 minutes Cooking time: 15 minutes Servings: 4

Ingredients:
- 1 cup pecans
- ¼ cup brown sugar
- 1 teaspoon vanilla extract
- ¼ teaspoon ground cardamom
- ½ teaspoon ground clove
- ¼ cup of water

Directions:

15. Mix up together pecans, brown sugar, vanilla extract, ground cinnamon, and ground clove. Shake the mixture well and transfer it into the instant pot.
16. Set Saute mode and cook pecans for 5 minutes. Stir them constantly.
17. Then add water and mix up carefully.
18. Set manual mode and close the lid.
19. Cook pecans for 8 minutes. Then use quick pressure release.
20. Meanwhile, preheat oven to 365F.
21. Line the tray with baking paper.

22. Drain the water from pecans and transfer nuts on the tray.
23. Place them in the preheated oven and cook for 2-3 minutes.
24. Chill the pecans and store them in the paper bags.

Nutrition value/serving: calories 57, fat 2, fiber 0.3, carbs 9.6, protein 0.4

Spicy Edamame Snack

Prep time: 10 minutes Cooking time: 11 minutes Servings: 6

Ingredients:
- 1 cup edamame beans
- 1 teaspoon minced garlic
- 1 tablespoon almond butter
- ½ teaspoon cayenne pepper
- 1 tablespoon sesame seeds
- ¼ cup of soy sauce
- ¼ teaspoon salt
- ½ teaspoon brown sugar
- 1 cup water, for cooking

Directions:
13. Pour water in the instant pot. Add edamame beans and salt.
14. Close and seal the lid. Set Manual mode and cook beans for 6 minutes. Then use quick pressure release.
15. Meanwhile, mix up together minced garlic, cayenne pepper, sesame seeds. brown sugar, and soy sauce.
16. Transfer cooked edamame beans in the bowl.

17. Toss almond butter in the instant pot and melt it on Saute mode.
18. Add soy sauce mixture and bring to boil it (approximately 5 minutes).
19. Then open the lid and chill the sauce to room temperature.
20. Pour the sauce over the edamame beans and mix up well.

Nutrition value/serving: calories 89, fat 4.3, fiber 2.6, carbs 7.5, protein 5.6

Tempeh Potato Wraps

Prep time: 10 minutes Cooking time: 3 hours Servings: 6

Ingredients:
- 1 potato, peeled, chopped
- 8 oz tempeh, chopped
- 1 teaspoon brown sugar
- 1 tablespoon apple cider vinegar
- 1 tablespoon of liquid smoked
- 2 tablespoons tamari
- ½ teaspoon ground black pepper
- 1 tablespoon coconut oil
- 1 cup of water
- 6 corn tortillas

Directions:
12. Place tempeh and chopped potato in the instant pot.
13. Add brown sugar, apple cider vinegar, liquid smoke, tamari, ground black pepper, coconut oil, and water.
14. Close the lid and set slow cook mode.
15. Cook the mixture for 3 hours.
16. Then open the lid, mix up the ingredients.

17. Fill the tortillas with cooked tempeh mixture and wrap them.

Nutrition value/serving: calories 173, fat 7.1, fiber 2.2, carbs 20.2, protein 9.6

Vegan Nuggets

Prep time: 10 minutes Cooking time: 6 minutes Servings: 8

Ingredients:
- ½ cup panko bread crumbs
- 1 tablespoon turmeric
- 4 oz rolled oats
- 1 onion, diced
- 1 tablespoon olive oil
- ½ teaspoon ground black pepper
- 1 teaspoon salt
- 1 tablespoon coconut milk
- 1 cup chickpeas, canned
- 1 tablespoon tomato sauce
- ½ cup water for cooking

Directions:
13. Preheat instant pot on Saute mode.
14. When it is hot, add olive oil and diced onion.
15. Cook it for 3-4 minutes, stir from time to time.

16. When the onion is soft, transfer it in the food processor.
17. Add rolled oats, ground black pepper, salt, coconut milk, canned chickpeas, and tomato sauce.
18. Blend the mixture until smooth.
19. In the separated bowl, mix up together turmeric and panko bread crumbs.
20. Make the medium size nuggets from the chickpea mixture.
21. Then coat nuggets in the panko bread mixture.
22. Pour water in the instant pot and insert rack.
23. Place instant pot pan on the rack and put nuggets inside it.
24. Close and seal the lid.
25. Set manual mode (high pressure) and cook "nuggets" for 3 minutes.
26. Then use quick pressure release.
27. Chill the cooked snack till the room temperature.

Nutrition value/serving: calories 200, fat 5.1, fiber 6.7, carbs 31.7, protein 7.9

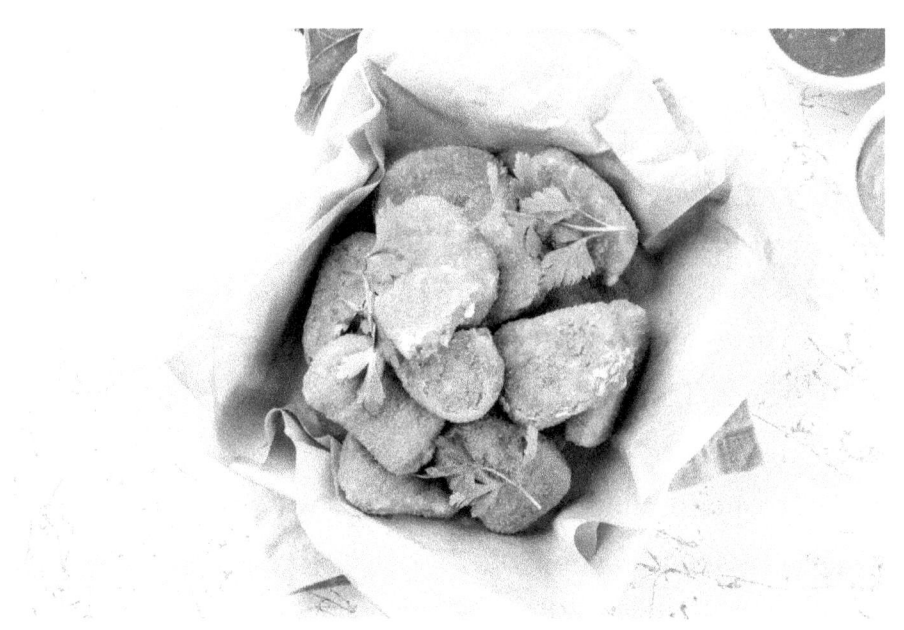

Crunchwrap Supreme

Prep time: 15 minutes Cooking time: 10 minute Servings: 4

Ingredients:
- 5 oz tofu, chopped
- 1 tablespoon olive oil
- 1 teaspoon taco seasoning
- 1 tablespoon salsa sauce
- 2 tablespoons queso sauce
- 4 burrito size tortillas
- 1/3 cup tortilla chips
- ½ cup black beans, canned
- 1 avocado, peeled, cored
- 1 tomato, chopped
- 1 teaspoon coconut oil

Directions:
18. Pour olive oil in the instant pot and preheat it on Saute mode.
19. Add chopped tofu and sprinkle it with taco seasoning.
20. Cook it on saute mode for 2 minutes. Stir it.
21. Then mash the avocado.
22. Spread the burrito tortillas with mashed avocado.

23. After this, add salsa sauce, cooked tofu, chopped tomatoes, and black beans.
24. Repeat the same steps with all burrito tortillas.
25. Place tortilla chips on the top of black beans and wrap burrito tortillas.
26. Toss coconut oil in the instant pot, melt it on Saute mode and add wrapped burrito tortillas.
27. Cook them for 3 minutes from each side.

Nutrition value/serving: calories 518, fat 26.1, fiber 9.6, carbs 58.4, protein 14.4

Spring Rolls

Prep time: 15 minutes Cooking time: 4 minutes Servings: 6

Ingredients:
- ¼ cup red cabbage, shredded
- 2 oz fresh parsley, chopped
- 1 cup mushrooms, chopped
- 1 carrot, cut into wedges
- 1 tablespoon fish sauce
- 1 teaspoon paprika
- 1 tablespoon lemon juice
- ¼ teaspoon lime zest
- ½ teaspoon chili flakes
- 6 spring roll wraps
- 1 cup water, for cooking

Directions:

13. In the mixing bowl, mix up together shredded red cabbage, fresh parsley, chopped mushrooms, carrot, fish sauce, paprika, lemon juice, lime zest, and chili flakes.

14. Fill the spring roll wraps with cabbage mixture. Wrap the spring roll wraps.

15. Pour water in the instant pot, insert steamer rack inside.
16. Place prepared spring rolls on the steamer rack.
17. Close and seal the lid.
18. Set Manual mode (high pressure) and cook the meal for 4 minutes.
19. Then allow natural pressure release for 5 minutes.

Nutrition value/serving: calories 22, fat 0.2, fiber 1.9, carbs 4.5, protein 2

Delicious Lettuce Wraps

Prep time: 10 minutes Cooking time: 4 minutes Servings: 4

Ingredients:
- 4 lettuce leaves
- 3 oz vegan Parmesan, grated
- 1 cucumber, chopped
- 1 tablespoon chives, chopped
- 8 oz tempeh, chopped
- 1 tablespoon Italian seasoning
- 3 tablespoons tomato sauce
- ¼ cup tomato juice
- 1 teaspoon brown sugar
- 1/3 cup turnip, chopped

Directions:
11. In the instant pot, combine together chopped tempeh, Italian seasoning, tomato sauce, tomato juice, brown sugar, and turnip.
12. Mix up the mixture, close and seal the instant pot lid.
13. Cook it on Manual for 4 minutes; use quick pressure release.

14. After this, mix up together grated Parmesan chopped cucumber, and chives.
15. Place the mixture on the lettuce leaves.
16. Chill the tempeh mixture till the room temperature.
17. Transfer it over the vegetables and wrap the lettuce leaves.

Nutrition value/serving: calories 209, fat 7.3, fiber 0.9, carbs 15.7, protein 20.1

Garlic Toasts

Prep time: 5 minutes Cooking time: 2 minutes Servings: 4

Ingredients:
- 4 grey bread slices
- 1 tablespoon minced garlic
- 1 tablespoon olive oil

Directions:
13. Preheat instant pot. When it is hot, add olive oil.
14. Then add bread slices and cook them on Saute mode for 1 minute from each side.
15. Remove the bread slices from the instant pot and rub with minced garlic from each side.
16. Serve the toasts warm.

Nutrition value/serving: calories 153, fat 8, fiber 0, carbs 17.7, protein 3.1

Quinoa Sandwich

Prep time: 10 minutes Cooking time: 5 minutes Servings: 2

Ingredients:

- 4 bread slices
- ¼ cup quinoa
- ½ cup of water
- 1 teaspoon salt
- 1 tablespoon vegan mayonnaise
- ½ teaspoon paprika
- 1 oz micro greens

Directions:

13. Place water, salt, and quinoa in the instant pot.
14. Close and seal the lid.
15. Set manual mode and cook quinoa for 5 minutes. Then allow natural pressure release.
16. Open the lid and transfer it in the mixing bowl.
17. Add paprika and vegan mayonnaise. Mix it up.
18. Spread 2 bread slices with quinoa mixture. Add microgreens and cover with the remaining bread slices to get sandwiches.

Nutrition value/serving: calories 148, fat 3.7, fiber 2.7, carbs 24.1, protein 5

Crispy Chickpea

Prep time: 10 minutes Cooking time: 57 minutes Servings: 4

Ingredients:
- 7 oz chickpeas
- 4 cups of water
- 1 teaspoon salt
- 1 tablespoon Taco seasoning
- 1 tablespoon olive oil
- 1 teaspoon ground black pepper

Directions:

12. Place chickpeas, salt, and water in the instant pot. Close and seal the lid.
13. Cook the chickpeas on Manual mode (high pressure) for 50 minutes.
14. Then use quick pressure release and open the lid.
15. Drain water and dry the chickpeas with the help of the paper towel.
16. Then add olive oil, Taco seasoning, and ground black pepper.
17. Mix the mixture up.

18. Cook it on Saute mode for 7 minutes. Stir it from time to time.

19. Chill the cooked chickpeas little bit and transfer in the serving bowl.

Nutrition value/serving: calories 219, fat 6.5, fiber 8.8, carbs 31.9, protein 9.6

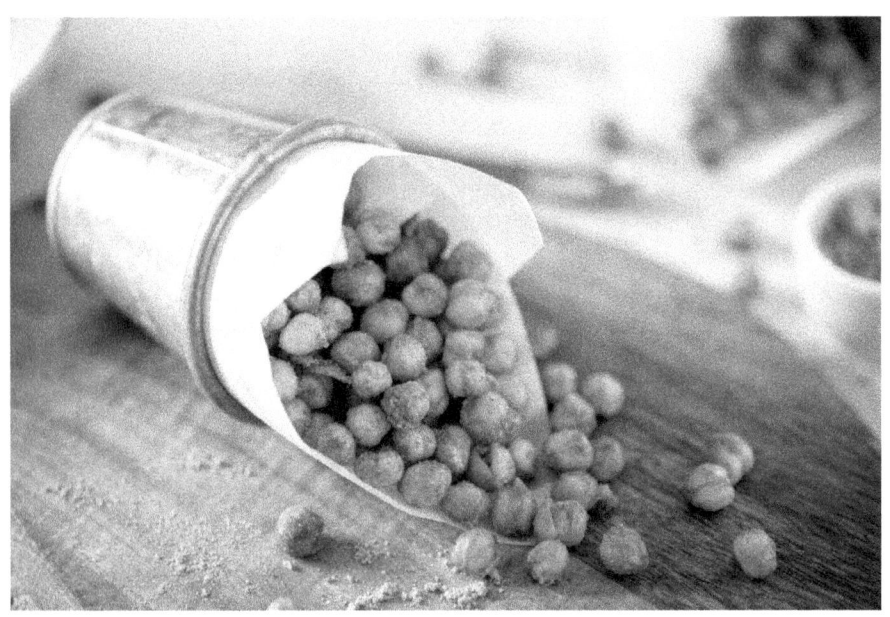

Turkish Vegan Borek

Prep time: 10 minutes Cooking time: 16 minutes Servings: 6

Ingredients:
- 3 cups spinach, chopped
- 1 tablespoon coconut oil
- 1 teaspoon salt
- 1 teaspoon ground black pepper
- 4 oz phyllo dough

12. Place spinach, salt, and coconut oil in the instant pot.
13. Cook the ingredients on Saute mode for 10 minutes. Stir them from time to time.
14. Then transfer spinach on the phyllo dough and roll it.
15. Place the rolled dough in the instant pot and cook it for 3 minutes from each side on Saute mode.
16. The cooked borek should have a light brown color.
17. When borek is cooked, cut it into the serving pieces.

Nutrition value/serving: calories 80, fat 3.5, fiber 0.8, carbs 10.7, protein 1.8

Vegan Jerky

Prep time: 20 minutes Cooking time: 3 hours Servings: 2

Ingredients:
- 5 oz tempeh, cut into wedges
- 1 teaspoon BBQ sauce
- 1 teaspoon soy sauce
- 1 teaspoon lemon juice
- 1 teaspoon chili pepper
- ½ teaspoon brown sugar
- 1 teaspoon olive oil

Directions:

11. Make the marinade: in the bowl whisk together BBQ sauce, soy sauce, lemon juice, chili pepper, brown sugar, and olive oil.
12. Place tempeh wedges in the marinade and marinate them for 15 minutes.
13. After this, dry the tempeh wedges with the help of the paper towel and transfer in the instant pot.
14. Close the lid and cook jerky on slow cooker mode for 3 hours.

Nutrition value/serving: calories 167, fat 10, fiber 0.2, carbs 8.9, protein 13.4

Carrot "Dogs"

Prep time: 15 minutes Cooking time: 4 minutes Servings: 4

Ingredients:
- 4 hot dog buns
- 4 teaspoons mustard
- 4 teaspoon ketchup
- 4 carrots, peeled
- 1 tablespoon fish sauce
- 1 teaspoon liquid smoke
- 2 cups of water

Directions:
13. Pour water in the instant pot.
14. Add carrots, fish sauce, and liquid smoke. Close and seal the
lid.
15. Cook carrots on Manual mode for 4 minutes. Then make
quick pressure release.
16. Open the lid and let carrots stay in liquid for at least 10 minutes.

17.   Then fill hot dog buns with carrots, add ketchup and mustard.

Nutrition value/serving: calories 187, fat 3, fiber 2, carbs 33.6, protein 4.6

Gyros

Prep time: 15 minutes Cooking time: 15 minutes Servings: 4

Ingredients:
- 1 cucumber, grated
- 6 oz firm tofu, chopped
- 2 tablespoons lime juice
- 1 teaspoon minced garlic
- 1 teaspoon rice vinegar
- 1 tablespoon dried dill
- 1 cup lettuce, chopped
- 1 red onion, sliced
- 4 pitas or corn tortillas
- 4 Portobello mushrooms
- 1 tablespoon olive oil
- 1 teaspoon ground black pepper
- ½ teaspoon chili pepper
- ½ teaspoon ground coriander
- 1 tablespoon liquid smoke

Directions:

13. Cut Portobello mushrooms into the wedges and sprinkle them with olive oil, ground black pepper, chili pepper, ground coriander, and liquid smoked.

14. Transfer the mushrooms in the instant pot.

15. Cook them on Saute mode for 15 minutes. Stir them from time to time.

16. Meanwhile, put in the blender: tofu, cucumber, lime juice, minced garlic, rice vinegar, and dried dill.

17. Blend the ingredients until you get a smooth mixture.

18. Spread pitas with the smooth tofu mixture, add lettuce, and sliced red onion.

19. When the mushrooms are cooked, transfer them over the red onion.

20. Wrap pitas.

Nutrition value/serving: calories 275, fat 6.2, fiber 4.1, carbs 44.2, protein 13.1

Herbed Tomato

Prep time: 5 minutes Cooking time: 20 minutes Servings: 4

Ingredients:
- 4 tomatoes
- 1 oz fresh cilantro, chopped
- 3 garlic cloves, peeled
- 1 teaspoon ground black pepper
- ½ teaspoon salt
- 1 teaspoon oregano
- 1 tablespoon apple cider vinegar
- 1/3 cup water

Directions:
8. Cut tomatoes into the halves and place in the instant pot.
9. Add fresh cilantro, garlic cloves, ground black pepper, salt, oregano, apple cider vinegar, and water.
10. Close the lid and cook the meal on Saute mode for 20 minutes. Stir it from time to time.
11. Chill the tomatoes to the room temperature and transfer into the serving bowl.

Nutrition value/serving: calories 30, fat 0.4, fiber 2, carbs 6.4, protein 1.5

Lentils Crackers

Prep time: 10 minutes Cooking time: 10 minutes Servings: 8

Ingredients:
- 1 cup green lentils, cooked
- ½ cup flax meal
- 1 teaspoon ground black pepper
- 1 teaspoon salt
- 1 teaspoon dried parsley
- 4 teaspoons coconut oil

Directions:

14. Blend lentils until you get the smooth mixture and transfer them in the mixing bowl.
15. Add flax meal, ground black pepper, salt, dried parsley, and coconut oil.
16. Mix it up and knead the non-sticky dough.
17. Roll up the lentils dough with the help of the rolling pin.
18. Then make medium size crackers from the dough. Use the cracker cutter for this step.
19. Preheat instant pot on Saute mode.

20. Place the layer of the crackers inside and cook them for 1.5- 2 minutes from each side or until they start to be crunchy.
21. Repeat the same step with all prepared crackers.
22. Chill the crackers well and store them in the paper bags.

Nutrition value/serving: calories 135, fat 5, fiber 9.4, carbs 16.6, protein 7.7

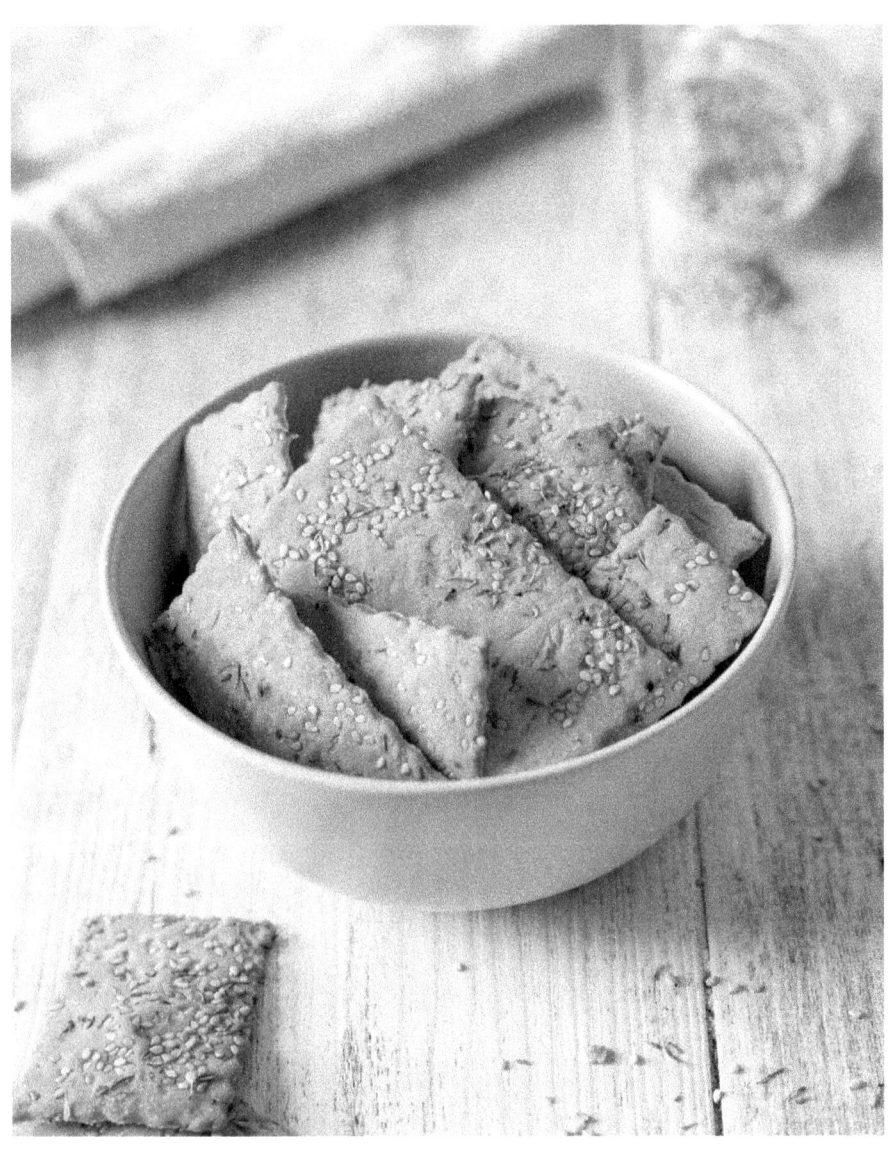

Eggplant Rolls

Prep time: 10 minutes Cooking time: 10 minutes Servings: 4

Ingredients:
- 1 large eggplant, trimmed
- 1 tablespoon minced garlic
- ½ cup arugula, chopped
- 1 tablespoon olive oil
- 1 tablespoon vegan ricotta
- 1 tablespoon peanuts, chopped

Directions:
14. Cut eggplants lengthwise slices. Sprinkle them with salt if desired.
15. Then preheat instant pot on Saute mode well.
16. Add olive oil.
17. Place eggplant slices in the instant pot and cook them for 2 minutes from each side.
18. Meanwhile, mix up together vegan ricotta, peanuts, arugula, and minced garlic.
19. Chill the eggplant slices well.
20. Then spread them with ricotta mixture and roll.
21. Secure rolls with the toothpicks.

Nutrition value/serving: calories 99, fat 6.8, fiber 4.4, carbs 9, protein 2.6

Mushroom Bruschetta

Prep time: 10 minutes Cooking time: 15 minutes Servings: 5

Ingredients:
- 5 bruschetta bread slices
- 1 cup mushrooms, sliced
- 1 yellow onion, sliced
- ½ cup coconut cream
- 1 teaspoon olive oil
- 1 teaspoon salt

Directions:
13. Place sliced onion and mushrooms in the instant pot.
14. Add olive oil and salt.
15. Cook the vegetables on Saute mode for 5 minutes. Mix them up from time to time.
16. After this, add coconut cream. Mix up again and close the lid.
17. Cook the mushroom mixture for 10 minutes on Saute mode.
18. When the time is over, open the lid and chill the cooked meal little.

19. Place mushrooms mixture over the bruschetta bread slices.

Nutrition value/serving: calories 255, fat 16.7, fiber 1.1, carbs 19.8, protein 6.2

BBQ Cauliflower Florets

Prep time: 15 minutes Cooking time: 15 minutes Servings: 2

Ingredients:
- 1 cup cauliflower florets
- 4 tablespoons BBQ sauce
- 1 teaspoon turmeric
- 1 teaspoon paprika
- 1 teaspoon cayenne pepper
- ¼ cup of water
- 1 teaspoon olive oil

Directions:
13. Place cauliflower florets in the bowl.
14. Add BBQ sauce, turmeric, paprika, cayenne pepper, olive oil, and water.
15. Carefully mix up the cauliflower and leave it for 5-10 minutes to marinate.
16. Then transfer it in the instant pot, add all the remaining BBQ sauce mixture.
17. Saute the cauliflower for 10-15 minutes or until it is cooked. Stir it time to time with the help of the wooden spatula.

18. Chill the cooked snack till the room temperature and then transfer in the serving bowl or serve in the closed glass vessel in the fridge up to 2 days.

Nutrition value/serving: calories 89, fat 2.9, fiber 2.3, carbs 15.8, protein 1.3

Asparagus Pastries

Prep time: 15 minutes Cooking time: 10 minutes Servings: 8

Ingredients:
- 8 oz vegan puff pastry
- 11 oz asparagus
- 1 tablespoon olive oil
- ½ teaspoon salt
- 1 teaspoon dried oregano
- 1 cup water, for cooking

Directions:
17. Roll up the puff pastry with the help of the rolling pin.
18. Then cut it into the strips.
19. Mix up together salt, dried oregano, and olive oil.
20. Spread the puff pastry strips with the oregano mixture.
21. Then wrap the strips around the asparagus.
22. Pour water in the instant pot. Insert steamer rack
23. Line it with the baking paper.
24. Place wrapped asparagus over it.
25. Close and seal the lid.
26. Set Manual mode (high pressure) and cook pastries for 10 minutes. Then use quick pressure release.

27. Chill the cooked pastries well before serving.

Nutrition value/serving: calories 182, fat 12.7, fiber 1.3, carbs 14.6, protein 3

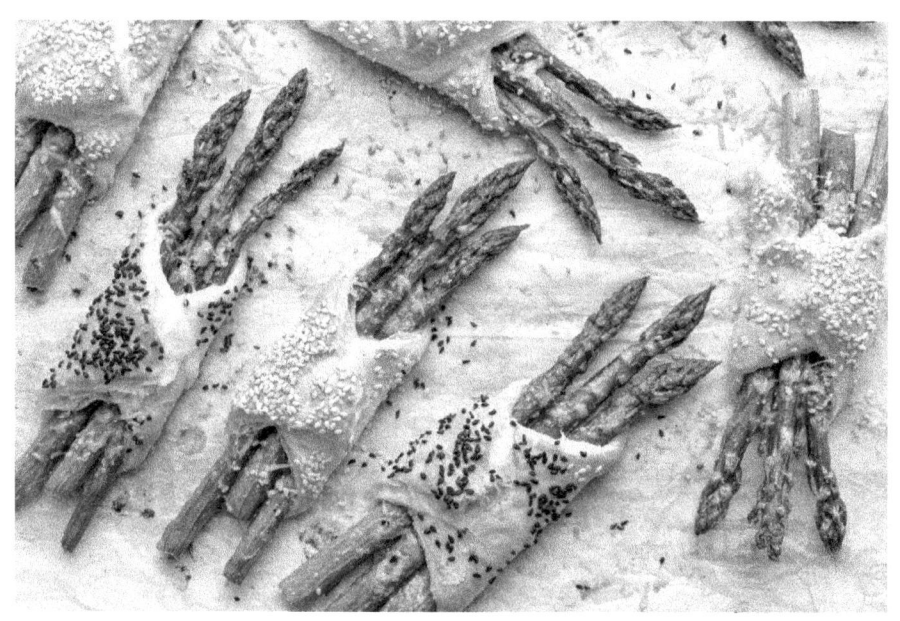

Cocktail Balls

Prep time: 10 minutes Cooking time: 10 minutes Servings: 4

Ingredients:
- 1 cup mashed potato
- ¼ cup panko bread crumbs
- 1 teaspoon salt
- 3 tablespoons flax meal
- 1 tablespoon fresh parsley, chopped
- ½ onion, grated
- 1 tablespoon avocado oil

Directions:
17. Mix up together mashed potato, panko bread crumbs, salt, flax meal, parsley, and grated onion.
18. When you get a homogenous mixture, make medium size balls. Do it with the help of 2 spoons or fingertips.
19. Preheat avocado oil in the instant pot
20. Add potato balls and roast them on Saute mode for 2 minutes from each side.
21. Dry the cooked balls with the help of the paper towel and transfer on the serving plate. Put the toothpicks inside.

Nutrition value/serving: calories 119, fat 4.9, fiber 3.1, carbs 16.8, protein 3.3

Arugula Puffs

Prep time: 15 minutes Cooking time: 4 minutes Servings: 4

Ingredients:
- 7 oz phyllo dough
- 1 teaspoon olive oil
- 5 oz vegan Cheddar cheese, grated
- ½ cup arugula, chopped
- ½ teaspoon thyme

Directions:
13. Cut phyllo dough into 4 equel squares.
14. Then in the center of every phyllo square put grated cheese, chopped arugula, and thyme.
15. Wrap the phyllo squares in such a way to get the envelopes – arugula puffs.
16. Pour olive oil in the instant pot.
17. Preheat it well on Saute mode.
18. Then place phyllo envelops in the instant pot and cook them 3 minutes.
19. After this, flip the meal onto another side and cook for 1 minute.
20. Serve the arugula puffs warm.

Nutrition value/serving: calories 263, fat 10.5, fiber 2.6, carbs 33.2, protein 4.5

Beetroot Fold-Overs

Prep time: 15 minutes Cooking time: 30 minutes Servings: 6

Ingredients:
- 2 beetroots, trimmed
- 2 cups of water
- 6 oz vegan Parmesan, grated
- 1 teaspoon minced garlic
- 1 tablespoon scallions, chopped
- 1 tablespoon almond yogurt
- ¼ teaspoon smoked paprika
- 1/3 cup fresh parsley, chopped

Directions:

17. Place beetroots in the instant pot. Add water and close the lid.
18. Cook beetroots on Manual mode (high pressure) for 30 minutes.
19. Then allow natural pressure release for 10 minutes. Chill and peel the cooked beetroots.
20. In the mixing bowl, mix up together grated Parmesan, minced garlic, scallions, almond yogurt, smoked paprika, and chopped parsley.

21. Slice the beetroots.

22. Fill the beetroot slices with the cheese mixture and fold over every slice.

Nutrition value/serving: calories 106, fat 0.2, fiber 0.9, carbs 9.8, protein 12.3

Sweet Apple Wedges

Prep time: 15 minutes Cooking time: 5 minutes Servings: 4

Ingredients:
- 3 apples
- ¼ cup maple syrup
- ½ teaspoon ground ginger
- ½ teaspoon ground cinnamon
- ½ teaspoon cardamom
- 1 tablespoon brown sugar
- 1 tablespoon coconut oil

Directions:
24. Cut the apples into the halves and remove seeds.
25. Then cut the apples into 2 wedges more.
26. Preheat instant pot and toss coconut oil inside.
27. Add maple syrup, ground ginger, brown sugar, ground cinnamon, and ground cardamom.
28. Stir the mixture until homogenous.
29. Add apple wedges and coat them well.
30. Saute the fruits for 3 minutes. Then switch off the instant pot and let apple wedges rest for at least 10 minutes before serving.

Nutrition value/serving: calories 179, fat 3.8, fiber 4.3, carbs 39.1, protein 0.5

Candied Pecans

Prep time: 5 minutes Cooking time: 5 minutes Servings: 5

Ingredients:
- 1 cup pecans
- ¼ cup of water
- ¾ cup maple syrup
- 1 teaspoon ground cinnamon
- 1 tablespoon brown sugar
- 3 tablespoons white sugar
- ¼ teaspoon salt

Directions:
22. Cut the pecans into halves.
23. Then place them in the instant pot.
24. Add maple syrup, ground cinnamon, and brown sugar.
25. Mix up the pecans and cook them on Saute mode 3 minutes. Stir them constantly.
26. When sugar is melted, switch off the instant pot.
27. Add salt and white sugar. Mix up pecans well.
28. Place the cooked pecans in the paper envelopes for snacks.

Nutrition value/serving: calories 359, fat 21.1, fiber 2.9, carbs 44.9, protein 2.7

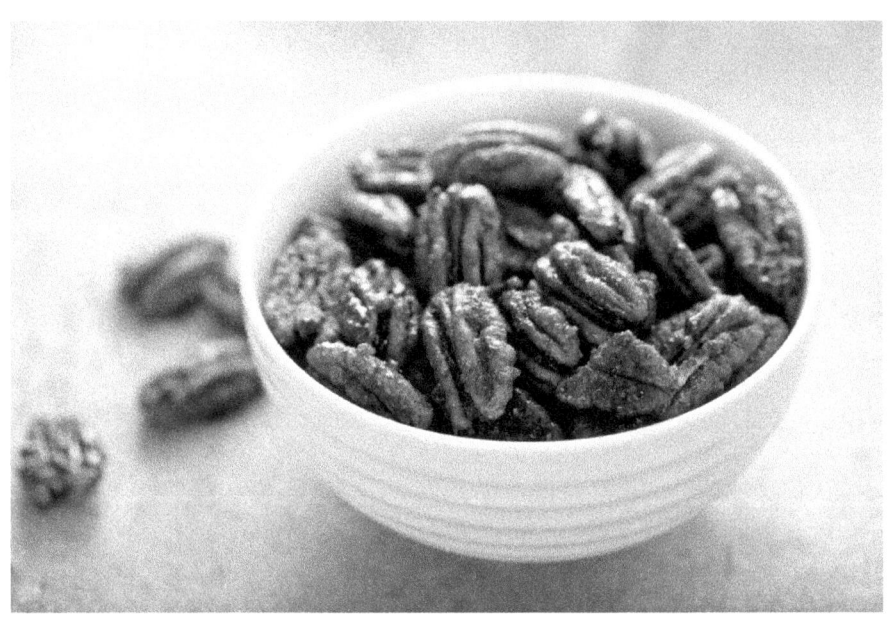

Buffalo Brussel Sprouts

Prep time: 10 minutes Cooking time: 10 minutes Servings: 4

Ingredients:
- 1 cup Brussel sprouts
- 5 tablespoons vegan Buffalo sauce
- 1 teaspoon olive oil
- 1 cup water, for cooking

Directions:
34. Pour water in the instant pot.
35. Add Brussel sprouts, close and seal the lid.
36. Cook the vegetables on Manual mode (high pressure) for 4 minutes.
37. Then use quick pressure release.
38. Drain water.
39. Pour olive oil in the instant pot.
40. Add Buffalo sauce and mix up well.
41. Cook Brussel sprouts on saute mode for 5 minutes. Stir them from time to time.
42. Chill the cooked appetizer to the room temperature before serving.

Nutrition value/serving: calories 29, fat 1.3, fiber 1.6, carbs 3.5, protein 0.8

Mushroom Pate

Prep time: 10 minutes Cooking time: 12 minutes Servings: 6

Ingredients:
- 1 shallot, diced
- 2 cups mushrooms, chopped
- 2 tablespoons almond butter
- 1 tablespoon avocado oil
- 1 teaspoon ground black pepper
- ½ teaspoon chili pepper
- 1 teaspoon salt
- 1 cup water, for cooking

Directions:

22. Put mushrooms and pour water in the instant pot.
23. Close and seal the lid. Cook mushrooms on manual mode for 8 minutes. Then use quick pressure release.
24. Open the lid and drain water.
25. Transfer the mushrooms in the food processor.
26. After this, pour avocado oil in the instant pot.
27. Preheat it on Saute mode.
28. Add diced shallot, ground black pepper chili pepper, and salt.

29. Saute shallot for 4 minutes or until it is light brown.
30. Then transfer it in the food processor too.
31. Add almond butter and blend the mixture well until you get soft pate.
32. Transfer cooked pate in the serving bowl.

Nutrition value/serving: calories 44, fat 3.4, fiber 1, carbs 2.7, protein 2

Cardamom Pineapple Sticks

Prep time: 15 minutes Cooking time: 5 minutes Servings: 4

Ingredients:
- 1 teaspoon ground cardamom
- 10 oz pineapple, cut into the sticks
- 2 tablespoon lemon juice
- ½ teaspoon brown sugar
- 1 tablespoon water
- ¼ teaspoon lime zest

Directions:
23. In the mixing bowl, mix up together ground cardamom, lemon juice, brown sugar, water, and lime zest.
24. Then place pineapple sticks in the cardamom liquid and coat well.
25. Let them marinate for 10 minutes.
26. Meanwhile, preheat the instant pot on Saute mode well.
27. Place the pineapple sticks in the instant pot and roast them on Saute mode for 1.5 minutes from each side.
28. Chill the cooked snack.

Nutrition value/serving: calories 40, fat 0.2, fiber 1.2, carbs 10.2, protein 0.5

Appetizer Quinoa Balls

Prep time: 15 minutes Cooking time: 15 minutes Servings: 6

Ingredients:
- 1 cup quinoa
- 3 tablespoons flax meal
- 1 teaspoon dried oregano
- ¼ cup onion, diced
- 1 teaspoon ground black pepper
- 2 tablespoons wheat flour
- ½ cup vegetable stock
- 1 teaspoon tomato paste
- 1 teaspoon salt
- ½ teaspoon chili flakes
- 1 cup of water

Directions:

24. Place quinoa and water in the instant pot. Close and seal the
lid.

25. Cook the quinoa on Manual mode for 5 minutes. Then use

quick pressure release. Transfer the quinoa in the mixing bowl.

26. Then place diced onion in the instant pot.
27. Add dried oregano, salt, tomato paste, chili flakes.
28. Saute the onions for 3 minutes. Mix up the onions and add them in the quinoa bowl.
29. Add flax meal, wheat flour, and ground black pepper.
30. Mix up the mixture.
31. Make the medium size bowls from quinoa mixture.
32. Then pour vegetable stock in the instant pot.
33. Insert trivet.
34. Place quinoa balls in the instant pot pan. Place the pan on the trivet.
35. Close and seal the lid.
36. Cook the quinoa balls for 5 minutes. Use quick pressure release.

37. Place the meal on the serving plate and sprinkle with the small amount of vegetable stock.

Nutrition value/serving: calories 135, fat 3.4, fiber 3.4, carbs 22.5, protein 5.2

Tofu Strips

Prep time: 5 minutes Cooking time: 5 minutes Servings: 4

Ingredients:
- 9 oz firm tofu
- 1 teaspoon miso paste
- 1 teaspoon tahini paste
- ¼ cup of water
- 1 teaspoon soy sauce
- 1 tablespoon balsamic vinegar
- 1 teaspoon olive oil
- 1 tablespoon fresh parsley, chopped

Directions:
22. Cut firm tofu into strips.
23. In the mixing bowl, mix up together miso paste, tahini paste, water, soy sauce, balsamic vinegar, and olive oil.
24. Coat tofu strips into the miso paste mixture.
25. Then preheat instant pot on Saute mode.
26. Place tofu stick and cook them for 1 minute from each side.
27. Transfer the tofu sticks on the serving plate and sprinkle with fresh parsley.

Nutrition value/serving: calories 67, fat 4.6, fiber 0.8, carbs 1.9, protein 5.7

Chickpea Slices

Prep time: 10 minutes Cooking time: 35 minutes Servings: 4

Ingredients:
- 4 flour tortillas
- ½ cup chickpeas, soaked
- 2 cups of water
- 1 teaspoon salt
- 1 tablespoon vegan mayonnaise
- 1 bell pepper, chopped

Directions:
21. Place tortillas and chickpeas in the instant pot.
22. Close and seal the lid.
23. Cook the chickpeas on Manual mode for 35 minutes. Use quick pressure release.
24. Drain the water and transfer the chickpeas in the blender.
25. Add salt, vegan mayonnaise, and bell pepper.
26. Blend the mixture.
27. Spread the flour tortillas with the blended chickpeas and roll them.

28. Slice the tortillas into small pieces and secure with toothpicks.

Nutrition value/serving: calories 162, fat 3.1, fiber 6.3, carbs 28.4, protein 6.5

Crunchy Oyster Mushrooms

Prep time: 15 minutes Cooking time: 15 minutes Servings: 3

Ingredients:
- 7 oz oyster mushrooms
- 1 tablespoon olive oil
- 1 teaspoon chili flakes
- ¼ cup bread crumbs
- 1 teaspoon apple cider vinegar
- 1 cup water, for cooking

Directions:
15. Place oyster mushrooms in instant pot pan.
16. Pour water in the instant pot and insert trivet.
17. Place pan with oyster mushrooms on the trivet and close the lid.
18. Seal the lid and cook mushrooms for 10 minutes.
19. After this, use quick pressure release.
20. Open the lid and drain water.
21. Chop the oyster mushrooms roughly and sprinkle with olive oil, chili flakes, and apple cider vinegar.

22. Mix up the mushrooms and let them for 10 minutes to marinate.
23. Then preheat instant pot on Saute mode.
24. Add oyster mushrooms and cook them for 4 minutes.
25. Stir the vegetables and sprinkle with bread crumbs. Mix up the mushrooms well.
26. Transfer them in the serving bowl.

Nutrition value/serving: calories 312, fat 5.2, fiber 7.5, carbs 44.3, protein 20.1

Jackfruit Coated Bites

Prep time: 15 minutes Cooking time: 5 minutes Servings: 4

Ingredients:
- 1 cup jackfruit, canned, drained
- ½ cup wheat flour
- 2 tablespoons soy sauce
- 2 tablespoons maple syrup
- 4 tablespoons agave syrup
- 1 teaspoon ground cumin
- ½ teaspoon salt
- 1 teaspoon paprika
- ½ teaspoon ground black pepper
- 1 teaspoon dried cilantro
- 1 teaspoon turmeric
- ½ cup olive oil

Directions:

23. In the mixing bowl, mix up together soy sauce, maple syrup, agave syrup, ground cumin, salt, and paprika. Whisk the mixture.

24. Place canned jackfruit in the soy mixture and mix up well. Leave it for 10 minutes to marinate.

25. Meanwhile, pour olive oil in the instant pot and preheat it on Saute mode.
26. In the separated bowl, combine together wheat flour, ground black pepper, cilantro, and turmeric.
27. Coat the jackfruit into the wheat mixture.
28. Place the coated pieces of jackfruit in the hot olive oil and cook them for 1 minute from each side or until light brown.
29. Dry the snack with the paper towel and transfer on the serving bowl.

Nutrition value/serving: calories 412, fat 257., fiber 1.,6 carbs 47, protein 3

Sofritas Tofu

Prep time: 5 minutes Cooking time: 5 minutes Servings: 4

Ingredients:
- 8 oz firm tofu, chopped
- ½ teaspoon cayenne pepper
- 1 teaspoon ground black pepper
- 1 teaspoon smoked paprika
- 1 teaspoon chili flakes
- ½ teaspoon salt
- ½ teaspoon brown sugar
- 1 tablespoon avocado oil
- 5 tablespoons vegan Adobo sauce

Directions:
23. Pour avocado oil in the instant pot. Add chopped tofu.
24. Cook it on Saute mode for 1 minute.
25. Sprinkle tofu with cayenne pepper, ground black pepper, smoked paprika, chili flakes, and salt. Mix up well and add sugar.
26. Stir it carefully and cook for 2 minutes.
27. Then add vegan Adobo sauce and mix up the meal well.
28. Cook it for 2 minutes more.

29. Transfer cooked sofritas tofu in the serving bowl.

Nutrition value/serving: calories 99, fat 2.9, fiber 1.1, carbs 13.6, protein 4.9

Garlic Pumpkin Seeds

Prep time: 5 minutes Cooking time: 10 minutes Servings: 6

Ingredients:
- 1 ½ cup pumpkin seeds
- 3 teaspoons garlic powder
- ½ teaspoon chipotle chili pepper
- 1 teaspoon salt
- 1 tablespoon olive oil

Directions:

26. Place pumpkin seeds in the instant pot.
27. Set Saute mode and cook them for 5 minutes. Stir pumpkin seeds every 1 minute.
28. After this, sprinkle the seeds with olive oil, chipotle chili pepper, salt, and garlic powder.
29. Mix up well and cook for 4 minutes more.
30. Then switch off the instant pot and let seeds rest for 1 minute.

Nutrition value/serving: calories 212, fat 18.2, fiber 1.6, carbs 7.3, protein 8.7

Flatbread

Prep time: 10 minutes Cooking time: 5 minutes Servings: 5

Ingredients:
- 1 cup wheat flour
- 1 teaspoon salt
- ¼ cup of water
- ¾ cup olive oil

Directions:

24. In the mixing bowl mix up together salt, water, and wheat flour.
25. Add olive oil and knead the soft and non-sticky dough.
26. Preheat instant pot on Saute mode well.
27. Meanwhile, cut dough into 5 buns and roll them up to make rounds.
28. Roast dough rounds in the instant pot for 1 minute from each side.
29. Cover cooked flatbreads with the cloth towel till serving.

Nutrition value/serving: calories 350, fat 30.5, fiber 0.7, carbs 19.1, protein 2.6

Polenta Fries

Prep time: 15 minutes Cooking time: 10 minutes Servings: 10

Ingredients:
- 1 cup polenta
- 3 cups almond milk
- 1 teaspoon salt
- 1 teaspoon ground black pepper
- 1 teaspoon dried cilantro
- ½ teaspoon ground cumin
- 1 tablespoon almond butter
- 1 tablespoon olive oil

Directions:

22. Place polenta in the instant pot. Add almond milk and salt.
23. Then add ground black pepper, dried cilantro, and ground cumin. Mix it up.
24. Close and seal the lid.
25. Cook polenta for 6 minutes on High-pressure mode. Allow natural pressure release for 10 minutes.
26. Open the lid and add almond butter. Mix up it well.

27. Transfer the polenta into the square pan and flatten well.
28. Let it chill until solid.
29. Then cut solid polenta onto 10 sticks.
30. Brush every stick with the olive oil.
31. Clean and preheat instant pot on Saute mode until hot.
32. Then cook polenta sticks for 1 minute from each side or until light brown.
33. Chill the snack before serving.

Nutrition value/serving: calories 244, fat 19.6, fiber 2.2, carbs 16.7, protein 3.2

Green Croquettes

Prep time: 15 minutes Cooking time: 5 minutes Servings: 4

Ingredients:
- 2 sweet potatoes, peeled, boiled
- 1 cup fresh spinach
- 1 tablespoons peanuts
- 3 tablespoons flax meal
- 1 teaspoon salt
- 1 teaspoon ground black pepper
- 1 tablespoon olive oil
- ½ teaspoon dried oregano
- ¾ cup wheat flour

Directions:
18. Mash the sweet potatoes and place them in the mixing bowl. Add flax meal salt, dried oregano, and ground black pepper.
19. Then blend the spinach with peanuts until smooth.
20. Add the green mixture in the sweet potato.
21. Mix up the mass.
22. Make medium size croquettes and coat them in the wheat flour.

23. Preheat instant pot on Saute mode well.
24. Add olive oil.
25. Roast croquettes for 1 minute from each side or until golden brown.
26. Dry the cooked croquettes with a paper towel if needed.

Nutrition value/serving: calories 155, fat 6.8, fiber 2.7, carbs 20.6, protein 4.4

Cigar Borek

Prep time: 10 minutes Cooking time: 5 minutes Servings: 6

Ingredients:
- 6 oz phyllo dough
- 8 oz vegan Parmesan, grated
- 1 tablespoon vegan mayonnaise
- 1 teaspoon minced garlic
- 1 tablespoon avocado oil

Directions:
20. In the mixing bowl, mix up together grated Parmesan, vegan mayonnaise, and minced garlic.
21. Then cut phyllo dough into triangles.
22. Spread the triangles with cheese mixture and roll in the shape of cigars.
23. Preheat avocado oil in the instant pot on Saute mode.
24. Place rolled "cigar" in the instant pot and cook them for 1-2 minutes or until they are golden brown.

Nutrition value/serving: calories 210, fat 2.6, fiber 0.7, carbs 23.1, protein 17.5

Flaked Clusters

Prep time: 10 minutes Cooking time: 4 minutes Servings: 4

Ingredients:
- 3 oz chia seeds
- ½ cup pumpkin seeds
- 1 cup coconut flakes
- 1/3 cup maple syrup
- 1 cup water, for cooking

Directions:

22. In the mixing bowl mix up together chia seeds, pumpkin seeds, coconut flakes, and maple syrup.
23. Then line the trivet with the baking paper.
24. Pour water in the instant pot. Insert lined trivet.
25. With the help of 2 spoons make medium size clusters (patties) from the coconut mixture and put them on the trivet.
26. Close and seal the lid.
27. Cook clusters for 4 minutes on High.
28. Then use quick pressure release and open the lid.

29. Transfer the cooked clusters on the plate and let them chill well.

Nutrition value/serving: calories 336, fat 21.2, fiber 9.8, carbs 32.7, protein 8.4

Chickpea Crackers

Prep time: 10 minutes Cooking time: 5 minutes Servings: 4

Ingredients:
- 1 cup chickpeas, cooked
- 1 teaspoon ground coriander
- 1 teaspoon cumin
- 1 teaspoon salt
- ½ teaspoon sesame seeds
- ¼ cup wheat flour
- 1 cup water, for cooking

Directions:

22. Put chickpeas, ground coriander, cumin, and salt in the blender.
23. Blend the mixture until smooth and transfer it in the mixing bowl.
24. Add wheat flour and sesame seeds. Mix it up with the help of a spoon.
25. Then line instant pot baking pan with baking paper.
26. Put chickpea mixture in the pan and flatten it well to get a thin layer.
27. Cut into square pieces.

28. Pour water in the instant pot and insert rack.
29. Place pan with chickpeas mixture on the rack. Close and seal the lid.
30. Cook the crackers for 3 minutes on High-pressure mode. Then use quick pressure release.
31. Open the lid, transfer crackers in the serving bowl and chill well.

Nutrition value/serving: calories 215, fat 3.4, fiber 9, carbs 36.6, protein 10.6

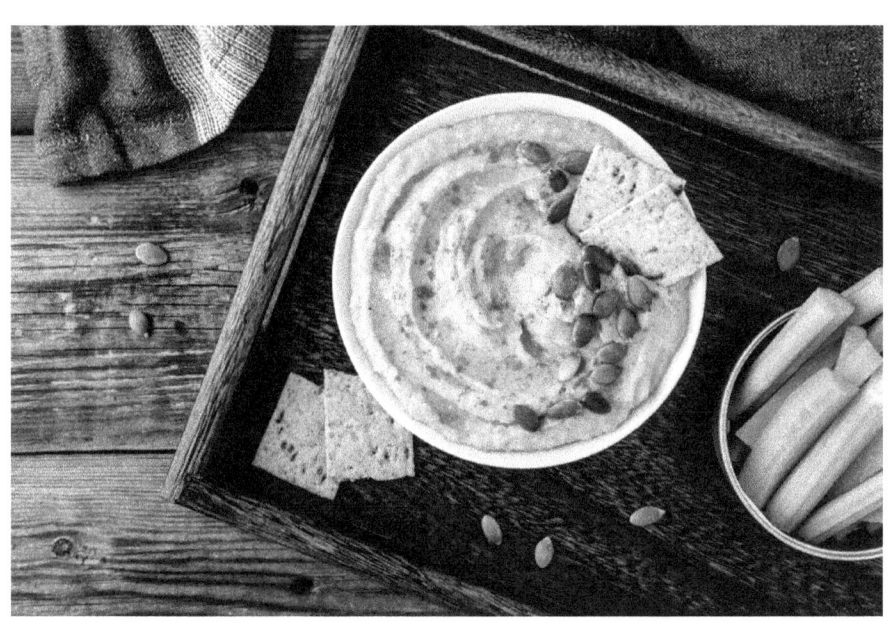

Eggplant Fries

Prep time: 15 minutes Cooking time: 5 minutes Servings: 4

Ingredients:
- 1 large eggplant
- 1 teaspoon salt
- 2 tablespoons wheat flour
- ½ teaspoon garlic powder
- 1 teaspoon ground black pepper
- 1 cup water, for cooking

Directions:
17. Trim the eggplant and cut it into wedges.
18. Then sprinkle with salt, garlic powder, and ground black pepper. Shake the vegetables well and leave for 5 minutes.
19. After this, coat every eggplant wedge with wheat flour.
20. Pour water in the instant pot, insert trivet.
21. Place pan on the trivet.
22. Transfer eggplant wedges in the pan.
23. Close and seal the instant pot lid.
24. Cook eggplants for 5 minutes on Manual mode (high pressure).

25. Use quick pressure release.

26. Dry the eggplant wedges with the paper towel gently.

Nutrition value/serving: calories 45, fat 0.3, fiber 4.3, carbs 10.3, protein 1.6

Crunchy Artichoke Hearts

Prep time: 15 minutes Cooking time: 10 minutes Servings: 2

Ingredients:
- 1/3 cup artichoke hearts, canned
- ½ cup panko bread crumbs
- ¼ cup almond milk
- 1 tablespoon flax meal
- 1 teaspoon paprika
- 2 tablespoons sesame oil

Directions:
16. Whisk together almond milk and flax meal.
17. Add paprika and stir well.
18. Then dip artichoke hearts into the almond milk mixture and coat in the panko bread crumbs.
19. Pour sesame oil in the instant pot.
20. Preheat it on saute mode.
21. Place coated artichoke hearts in the instant pot and cook them for 2 minutes from each side.

Nutrition value/serving: calories 329, fat 23.7, fiber 5.8, carbs 26.2, protein 6

Scallion Pancakes

Prep time: 10 minutes Cooking time: 5 minutes Servings: 4

Ingredients:
- ½ cup scallions, chopped
- 2 tablespoons flax meal
- 4 tablespoons water
- 1 teaspoon salt
- 1 potato, peeled, boiled
- 1 tablespoon olive oil
- 1 teaspoon ground black pepper

Directions:
23. Mix up together flax meal and water. Whisk it.
24. Add chopped scallions, salt, and ground black pepper.
25. After this, mash potato and add it in the scallions mixture.
26. Stir it well.
27. Make the balls from the mixture and press them to get pancake shape.
28. Pour olive oil in the instant pot. Preheat it on Saute mode.

29. Add scallions pancakes and cook them for 2 minutes from each side.

Nutrition value/serving: calories 83, fat 4.8, fiber 2.4, carbs 9.7, protein 1.9

Mushroom Arancini

Prep time: 10 minutes Cooking time: 6 minutes Servings: 8

Ingredients:
- ½ cup mushrooms, chopped, fried
- ½ cup of rice, cooked
- ½ onion, minced
- ¼ teaspoon minced garlic
- 4 oz vegan Parmesan, grated
- 3 tablespoons flax meal
- 5 tablespoons almond milk
- ¼ cup olive oil
- 1 cup bread crumbs

Directions:
20. Put chopped mushrooms, rice, minced onion, garlic, and grated cheese in the blender.
21. Blend the mixture for 30 seconds.
22. After this, transfer it in the mixing bowl.
23. In the separated bowl whisk together almond milk and flax meal.
24. Add the flax meal mixture in the rice mixture and stir well.

25. Pour olive oil in the instant pot and bring it to boil on Saute mode.
26. Meanwhile, make balls from the rice mixture and coat them in the bread crumbs well.
27. Place the mushroom balls in the hot olive oil and cook for 3 minutes or until light brown.
28. Dry the snack with the paper towel.

Nutrition value/serving: calories 230, fat 10.3, fiber 1.9, carbs 23.9, protein 9.4

Coated Heart of Palm

Prep time: 10 minutes Cooking time: 25 minutes Servings: 4

Ingredients:
- 1 cup heart of palm
- ¼ cup wheat flour
- ½ teaspoon salt
- 1 teaspoon maple syrup
- ½ teaspoon paprika
- ½ teaspoon soy sauce
- ¼ cup coconut flakes
- 2 tablespoon sesame oil

Directions:

23. Mix up together wheat flour, salt, paprika, and coconut flakes.
24. In the separated bowl, mix up together the heart of palm, maple syrup, and soy sauce. Stir gently.
25. Toss the heart of palm in the coconut flakes mixture and coat well.
26. Pour sesame oil in the instant pot and preheat it on Saute mode.

27. Cook coated heart of palm in the hot oil for 2 minutes. Then dry with the help of the paper towel.

28. Serve the snack with your favorite vegan sauce.

Nutrition value/serving: calories 122, fat 8.8, fiber 1.7, carbs 9.7, protein 2

Sweet Tofu Cubes

Prep time: 10 minutes Cooking time: 40 minutes Servings: 2

Ingredients:
- 6 oz firm tofu, cubed
- 1 teaspoon mustard
- 1 teaspoon olive oil
- 1 teaspoon apple cider vinegar
- ½ teaspoon maple syrup

Directions:
22. Place tofu in the instant pot.
23. Sprinkle it with mustard, olive oil, apple cider vinegar, and maple syrup.
24. Mix up the mixture well.
25. Close and seal the lid.
26. Cook tofu cubes for 2 minutes on High-pressure mode.
27. Then use quick pressure release.
28. Transfer the tofu cubes on the serving plate and sprinkle with the remaining gravy.
29. Insert a toothpick in every tofu cube.

Nutrition value/serving: calories 92, fat 6.4, fiber 1, carbs 3.2, protein 7.4

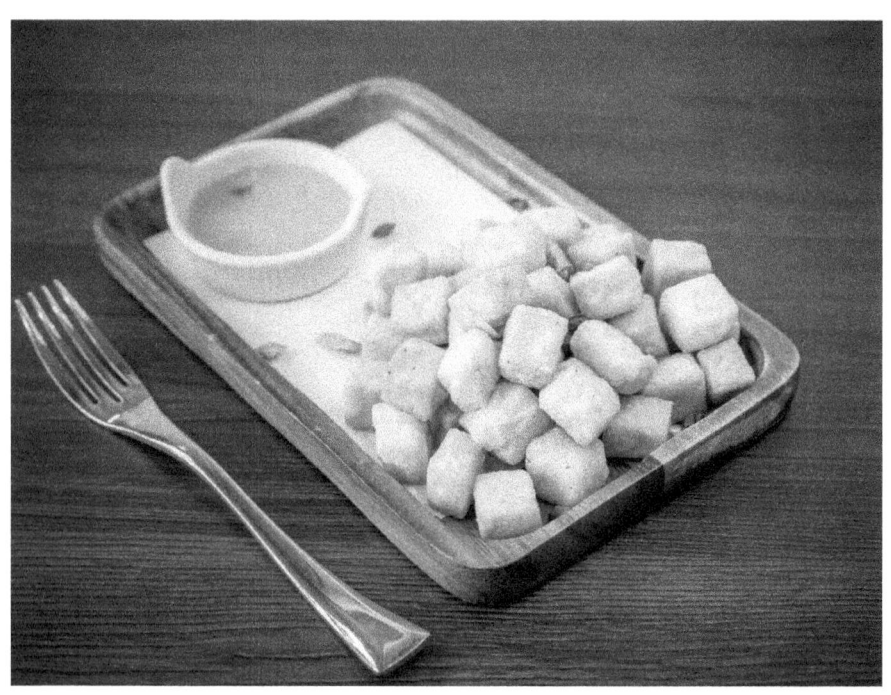

CPSIA information can be obtained
at www.ICGtesting.com
Printed in the USA
BVHW080953030321
601496BV00004B/791